Wisconsin's Early Home Remedies
by

Abing, Carriel
Allen, Mandy
Allen, Matt
Bader, Amy
Balachandran, Jay
Bartels, Aaron
Bast, Stacey
Baxter, Angie
Bowe, Erin
Brodbeck, Lindsay
Buchs, Stephen
Burgess, Cory
Butson, Heather
Chandler, Pat
Chandler, Tricia
Charles, David
Chase, Amy
Dehghan, Irene
Diedrichs, John
Draheim, Mahrya
Dreessens, Kathie
Egley, Marc
Eveland, Damian
Fowler, Benji
Fromader, Abby
Gardner, Chris
Gassman, Rhonda
Geasland, Kathy
Goke, Kiley
Haas, Bethany
Haas, Meagan
Hanson, Ken
Harrison, Mitchell
Hauser, Nick
Heiser, Lindsay
Honshel, Andrea
Jenny, Corey
Johnson, Kevin
Jonas, Victor
Jones, Shannon
Jones, Stephanie
Kies, Bethany
Kitto, Amanda
Klein, Ronnie
Kleisath, Beth
Klosterman, Tiffany
Kruser, Kelli
Lahey, Travis

Lange, Aaron
Larson, Beth
Leibfried, Ryan
Lynch, Jodi
McCabe, Sarah
MacKenzie, Daniel
MacKenzie, Matt
Mann, Brent
Maski, Manish
McFall, Amanda
McFall, Jenny Lolita
McKillip, Jenny
Mergen, Ryan
Moore, Amy
Moriarty, Carrie
Moyer, Christy
Mumm, Valerie
Murphy, Kelly
Nall, Tonya
Palmer, Brooke
Pink, Cory
Placko, Andy
Popp, Bryan
Ramaker, Brittney
Reuter, Jeremy
Richardson, Jill
Roskom, Kim
Sargent, Christy
Sharma, Ashlesha
Shea, Jill
Smidt, Sarah
Stint, Amy
Stoltz, Quintin
Swift, Troy
Thalmann, Ann
Thomas, Kelly
Timmerman, Stacy
Treige, Phyllis
Udelhofen, Jason
Uher, Jennifer
Van Natta, Shannon
Weier, Lindsay
Wetter, Denise
Wroblewski, Katie
Wunderlin, Jenny
Young, Sarah

* * * * * * * * * *

Although the authors have exhaustively researched all sources to ensure the accuracy and completeness of the information contained in this book, they assume no responsibility for errors, inaccuracies, ommisions, or any inconsistency herein. Any slights of people or organizations are unintentional. Readers should consult an attorney or accountant for specific applications to their individual publishing ventures.

QUIXOTE
PRESS
Bruce Carlson
R.R. #4, Box 33B
Blvd. Station
Sioux City, Iowa
51109

PRINTED
IN
U.S.A.

iii

DEDICATION

. . . . to our inventive relatives and friends

INTRODUCTION

We often reminisce about the "good old days." The past is a wonderful thing to explore.

This book brings together a collection of remedies which families used in earlier days when doctors were not always accessible, travel for health care was difficult, and people relied on their ingenuity and inventiveness at times of medical need. These home remedies were rediscovered by students of the Platteville Public Schools who enthusiastically interviewed their parents, grandparents, aunts, uncles, and friends to learn about the past and to find material for their stories.

I would like to thank not only the students who creatively wrote these anecdotal stories but also the teachers who encouraged them to go out into the community to discover its history. I would also like to thank the parents and all of the relatives and friends of the students who took the time to share their stories. This exploration into oral history has developed new friendships and helped to bond one generation to another.

We hope that this book adds to the body of knowledge about the history of Wisconsin and the people who live here. We also hope students feel a sense of accomplishment in seeing their contributions in print.

Lora DiMeglio
Gifted and Talented Specialist

Table of Contents

The reader is warned that these remedies have **not** necessarily been approved by medical practioneers.

The reader should not use these remedies instead of, or in addition to, usual contemporary medical procedures.

ACNE

Back in my grandfather's days, they hadn't invented CLEARASIL yet.

But pimples sure had been invented back then and they were the curse of the teenaged complexion just as they are today.

My grandfather, Ervin Christiansen, told my mother, Cheryl Larson, that a common practice in his community was to collect fresh urine and apply it to the pimples.

After that, the face would be gently rinsed off with water.

Grandfather Christiansen said that this would clear away the pimples in a couple of days.

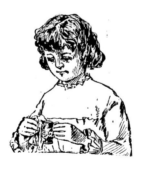

But I can tell you that I'm glad they invented Clearasil!

—Beth Larson

ASTHMA

My Aunt Lila from Platteville told me about an early home remedy that was supposed to get rid of asthma.

It sounds kind of gross to me, but what they used to do was to swallow a small fish. She said it worked well for them when she was little.

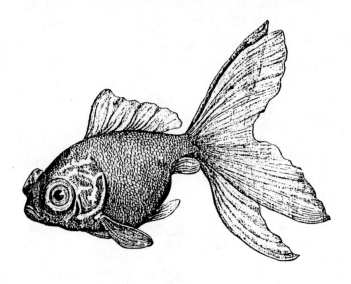

They didn't just eat a little fish like it was cooked and all. They had to swallow it whole.

—Ashlesha Sharma

CURE FOR BAD BLOOD

One time my great-grandma, Martha Dohse, made my mother drink a pint of sassafras tea every day for a full year.

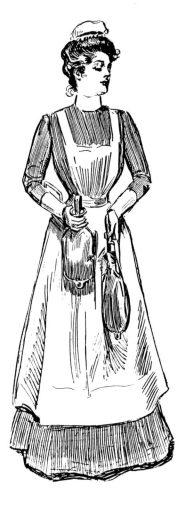

You see, my mother was supposed to have had bad blood, or anemia, and that was my grandmother's cure for bad blood.

Mother said she got pretty tired of that tea when she had to drink so much of it and had to do so every day for a year.

I know if I had to do that, I'd sure get tired of sassafras tea, whatever that is.

But, anyway, that sassafras tea must have worked 'cause my mother has good blood now.

—Amanda Kitto

BALDNESS

My grandpa was bald. Somewhere he came upon an article or book about how to cure baldness. So, he jumped right on that and faithfully followed the directions.

The instructions simply told him to rub the bald spot with onions in the morning and in the evening until it was red. Then he had to follow that up with rubbing it all over again with honey.

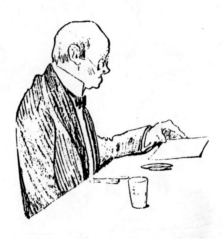

I really do have my doubts about that remedy since my Grandpa was bald until the day he died.

—Kelly Murphy

Beau Attracting

A couple of years ago I was talking to my great uncle at the Fliegel Family Frolic and he told me about how folks used to attract beaus back in the late 1800's.

You could concoct this remedy (or potion) at home with a simple mixture of vinegar and crushed dandelions.

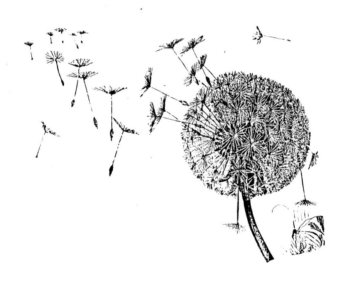

While my great uncle didn't tell me about if it would work or not, I kind of have my doubts about it.

—Phyllis Treige

(17)

BLACK EYES

When Murt Shea's brother bumped him in the eye with his elbow, his mother put beef steak on the eye.

The beef steak took the swelling down, and surprisingly enough, the eye didn't turn black and blue.

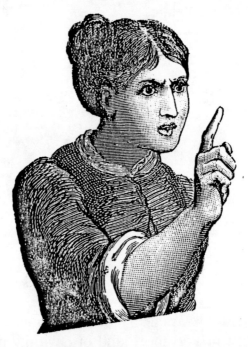

The boys also got a good lecture that day about being more careful to watch what they were doing so they didn't go around hurting one another.

—Jill Shea

It's hard to imagine a home remedy that is supposed to work for black eyes and scraped knees.

There doesn't seem to be a whole lot of connection between those two problems, but there must be since this remedy is supposed to be good for those two ailments.

My Aunt Lila told me that when she was a little girl they used to make a salve out of a mixture of lime, turmeric, and water.

This salve was supposed to be applied to the injured area.

Then, after the salve had dried out well, they would clean it off and put fresh salve on.

They would repeat this procedure until the knee or the eye was cured.

Aunt Lila said the remedy worked well for both problems.

—Ashlesha Sharma

BLEEDING

In the early days when a person got a cut and bled a lot, he often couldn't afford some of the things in the drugstore that were supposed to stop bleeding.

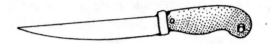

Dorothy Thiede of rural Wisconsin remembered hearing that when a cut wouldn't stop bleeding, one could use raw flour.

They would put the raw flour on the wound and then wrap it up real well and tight.

 They would let the flour do its thing for just a few minutes. Then they'd unwrap it again and wash the flour out of the area with nice warm water. They would do that washing very carefully so as not to get it bleeding again.

If the bleeding stayed stopped, they would then rewrap the wound until it healed.

—Ryan Mergen

Another cure for bleeding that couldn't be stopped is one that my father, Steve Kleisath, told me about. He knew some folks who used this and it worked well for them.

All the remedy amounts to is to put one tablespoon of cayenne pepper into a cup of hot water and to drink it.

This was supposed to stop the bleeding in about five minutes.

The first thing a person wonders about, of course, is how anyone could stand to down that much hot cayenne pepper.

My father told me that the theory was that if a person was bleeding badly he was probably hurting enough that he was in shock and so didn't even notice the hotness of the pepper. Then, by the time the person came out of shock, the taste of the pepper was about gone.

—Beth Kleisath

BLISTERS

My grandmother, Jane Hardy, told me about a blister remedy that has been in the Hardy family for many, many years.

Grandmother Hardy, in fact, used this remedy on my mother lots of times when she would get a blister from working or playing too hard.

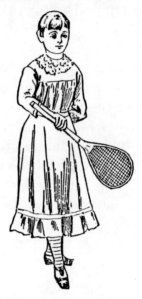

Grandmother would dab a little turpentine on the blister. Then she would put a thin piece of bacon fat on it.

Finally she'd wrap the area and leave the wrapping on overnight. By morning the blister would be almost healed.

—Marc Egley

BOILS

A man in his 90's who lived across the street from my grandma and grandpa told me about some home remedies from when he was a boy.

A really fun one is a remedy for boils. A boil is an inflamed and painful pus-filled swelling in the skin, and it has a hard center. It's caused by infection.

First, you have to apply a warm bread and milk poultice.

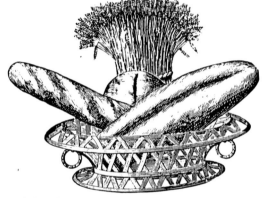

A poultice is a thick, hot, soft, moist mass applied to a sore or inflamed part of the body.

 To take the infection from a place, put a small jar in boiling water. Carefully take it out and put it over the boil. Cover with a cold, damp cloth. This creates a vacuum and the infection pops out!

—Abby Fromader

Here are five more remedies that are supposed to be good for boils.

(1) Apply a little Venice turpentine onto the boil.

(2) Apply a mixture of equal quantities of soap and brown sugar.

(3) Apply a little saffron in a white bread poultice.

(4) Apply a tablespoon of yeast in a glass of water, twice a day.

(5) Apply a plaster of honey and flour.

—Kelly Murphy

BRUISES

For a bruise or an earache, you can do what my mother's friend did for her husband. What you need is an onion and a bag. With a good sharp

knife, chop the onion and put it in the bag. Let it sit for three or four days. Then you can use it on the bruise or for an earache. It will take the pain away. It's better to start all that before the earache starts. That way you have it ready.

—Angie Baxter

BURNS & SCALDS

Here's a nice soothing home remedy that my Grandma Georgia Halverson from Soldiers Grove told me about.

Mix ground-up chalk with linseed or common olive oil such that you end up with a mixture about as thick as honey.

Then add vinegar so as to thin it back to the thickness of molasses.

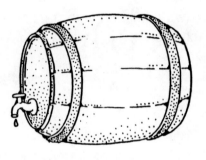

And since burns and scalds can hurt so badly, it is a good idea to apply the mixture to the area with a feather and keep renewing it from time to time.

—Kelly Murphy

Back when my grandparents were kids, burns were a painful and bothersome problem since there were so many stoves, fireplaces and bonfires to get burned on.

When my grandmother got a burn, her mother rubbed an aloe-vera plant on the spot.

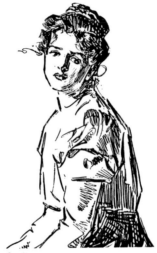

This stopped the pain and started the healing.

This remedy works very well, so the next time you get a burn, try this old-fashioned idea and save a trip to the doctor.

—Ronnie Klein

CAMPHOR CURES

This home remedy was brought to Wisconsin by my Grandma Bervelle Burback from Kentucky. It has been passed down from one generation to the next for a long time. My Great-Great-Grandmother Emily Cox told my Great-Grandmother Nellie Byrd about it.

There's probably been a bottle of this remedy tucked away in a cupboard or wardrobe somewhere in our family ever since it was part of the family.

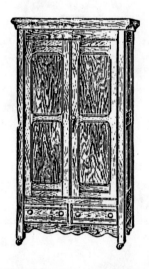

The remedy consists of cutting a cake of camphor gum into small chunks and putting it into a bottle of whiskey.

Just before you use it, give it a good shake to get it mixed well, and then immediately pour some out onto a rag, and then use it for whatever the ailment of the moment is.

This old family remedy isn't one that's just good for one thing, and that's it. It has a wide variety of applications and works well for all of them.

For example, if you fell off your horse and sprained a shoulder, out would come the old camphor and whiskey bottle.

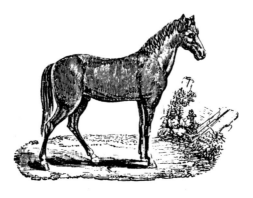

Rubbing a little bit of that stuff on the shoulder would have it fixed up in no time.

If you got a bruise, it was just as good for that, rubbing it on the bruise, or even just soaking it on there for a few minutes would get that bruise well on its way to recovery.

That camphor and whiskey was good for stomach cramps, cold sores, headaches and nausea.

Then, I suppose lots of family members would use it for other things, thinking that if it was good for all those, it must be good for other ailments also.

—Brittney Ramaker

CHAPPED LIPS

My grandma said to cure chapped lips all you need to do is to put a tablespoon of honey in with a few drops of rose water or lavender water.

Rubbing your lips with that will help a lot if you keep doing it several times throughout the day.

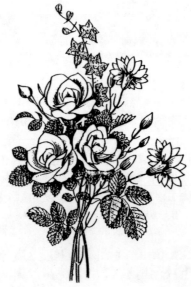

—Kelly Murphy

CHARLIE HORSES

When my Grandma Sharon Jones was growing up on a farm near Ellenboro, Wisconsin, the

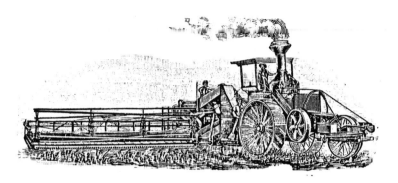

children were always getting charlie horses in their legs. Those things can be awfully painful, of course, and Grandma Jones had a home remedy that would offer some relief.

She'd put horse liniment on those painful legs to get rid of that pain.

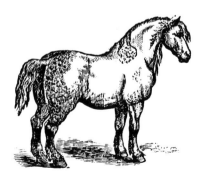

—Jennifer Uher

CHEST COLDS

My great-great aunt, Jo Esmay, uses a paste made of one tablespoon of dry yellow mustard and three tablespoons of flour mixed with a little water. She spreads some on a cloth and puts it on the chest. Another warm cloth is put on top of the first cloth.

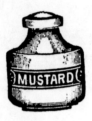

She leaves this on the chest until it gets warm. But she says you have to check it often because the skin can get red and hot.

—Travis Lahey

My great grandmother used to put a mustard pack on her children to sooth a cold.

To put on a mustard pack, you have to heat and dampen a cloth. Then you have to plaster it with a mustard mixture. Finally place it gently on the sick child's chest.

This will almost always help the child to breathe better; that is if he still wants to.

—Meagan Haas

When my Grandpa Eldon Lynch got a cold, as a child, his mother, Hortense, would warm up the wood stove.

When it got good and warm, she'd put a whole onion on the top to sort of bake.

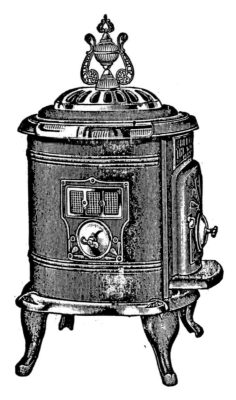

When the onion was good and baked, she made Eldon eat the whole thing. For the next few hours, he was just put to rest and was not allowed to roughhouse.

—Jodi Lynch

(33)

When my grandmother, Eileen Schneider, was young during the depression, money was scarce and she couldn't afford a doctor. So her mother used a home remedy for a child's cold so it didn't turn into pneumonia.

This was goose grease and turpentine. Great Grandma Ferris used goose grease on Grandma Eileen's chest, back, underarms, and the bottoms of her feet.

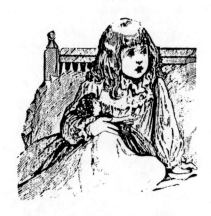

Then she dressed Grandma in warm pajamas or a nightgown, and threw two or three blankets on the bed to make her sweat. She used to sweat more than she does now.

Great Grandma Ferris did this every night for a week or two until the cold was gone. When Grandma got to feeling well, she would get to stop using the goose grease for a while.

—Kevin Johnson

Great Aunt Marie Parkenson from Darlington tells about how her mother would treat a cold there in her family.

"For a common chest cold, goose grease and turpentine was all that Mother needed. She'd mix these up to make an old-fashioned version of a vapor rub.

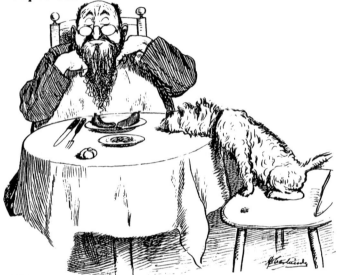

"Whenever she cooked a goose, the grease went into a pint jar. Turpentine got added later as the mixture was needed."

"That goose grease and turpentine was rubbed on the chest and neck. Then a flannel cloth got wrapped around the entire area."

—Aaron Bartels

My ancestors really went through a lot when they came down with a cold. In my grandpa's family, a really bad chest cold was treated with a glass of half whiskey and half hot water with a little lemon juice mixed in.

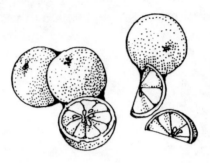

After a person drank that mess, he'd have to go to bed right away and cover up with lots of blankets to help with the "sweating out of the cold."

Other chest colds, not quite so serious, would be treated with goose grease and kerosene. They would add just enough kerosene to the grease to make a sort of salve. This was rubbed on the chest and didn't need to be covered with a cloth.

I had the goose grease and kerosene remedy tried on me once and it really did work, so maybe some of the others did, too.

—Heather Butson

My Grandma, Lilace Rouse, was born in January, 1914, in Benton, Wisconsin.

During her childhood, Grandma was exposed to several diseases and to several home remedies to combat those diseases. It was a close race sometimes as to which of the two was the worse.

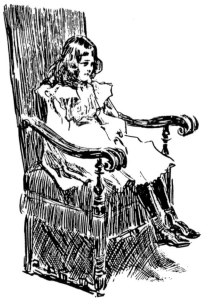

One thing they did to her was to fix a hot mustard pack for her whenever she took sick with a cold. It was something that Grandma could depend on.

Her mother would put hot mustard on her chest and cover the whole thing with a hot cloth. The mustard and the heat worked together to clear the congestion in her chest.

—Ann Thalmann

(37)

Sometimes these home remedies seem a little bit strange. My Grandmother Nana told me about how her cousin was in a camp while World War I was going on.

What people did there was to put their pants on over their head when they would go to sleep to protect them from the cold.

—Irene Dehghan

CHICKEN POX

Back when Anne-Marie Brodie was a young girl, she came down with the chicken pox.

As folks were apt to do back then, Anne-Marie's mother went to her own mother for some advice on what to do for the little girl.

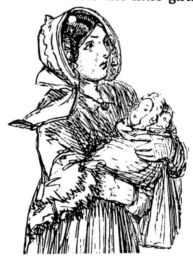

The grandmother told her daughter to have Annie-Marie bathe in a tub filled with liquid starch added to the bath water.

She said the tub had to be completely full so the little girl would be all the way up to her neck in it.

After two or three such soaking baths, Anne-Marie's chicken pox was all but gone.

—Jenny McKillip

(39)

COLD SORES

My grandpa, Bob Jones, got this old remedy from his mother.

She used to put earwax on cold sores. All she did was to take some ear wax and rub it on the cold sore to dry it up.

That all sounds kind of weird to me, but he said that it really works, and you can't taste the ear wax on your lip . . . very much, anyway.

—Jennifer Uher

This home remedy sounds like it would be awfully painful, but my mother told me that it not only works, but doesn't hurt a bit.

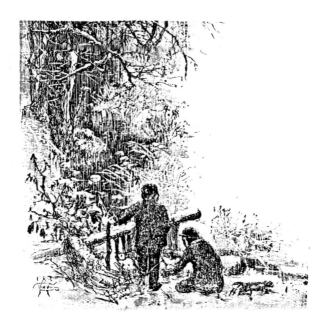

What it takes is one of those old-fashioned wooden matches and a person willing to take the chance that it won't hurt.

Someone will strike the match, blow it out, and while it is still hot, put it right on the cold sore.

The sulfur of the match is supposed to cure the cold sore.

—Amy Stint

(41)

Nancy Dieter of Platteville told me about this home remedy for cold sores. She said it is also good for chapped lips.

Nancy remembered that when she was a little girl she seemed to be always getting painful cold sores and chapped lips.

Nancy's family couldn't afford the storebought stuff you could get that was supposed to offer relief for those sort of problems.

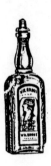 But her mother had a home remedy that she always used on the family.

This was kind of a gross remedy, but it did work.

What her mother would do was to smear a little ear wax on the lip or cold sore.

Nancy's mother claimed that not only was ear wax a whole lot cheaper than the store-bought stuff but would work better.

I know how painful chapped lips or cold sores can be, but I think that next time I get something like that I'll use CHAP-STICK instead of that ear wax treatment.

—Erin Bowe

(42)

COLIC

Babies that had colic were often given a little tea made from catnip.

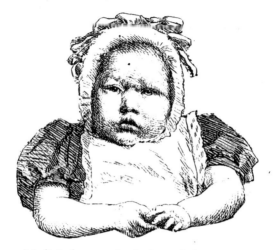

It wouldn't take a whole lot of that tea to really help them. It seemed that if you got even just a small amount down 'em, it would help.

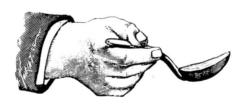

—Heather Butson

CONSTIPATION

For constipation of a baby, Hilda Chandler did the following:

Put a little Karo syrup in the baby's bottle or cup of milk and have the little one drink it. This will straighten the child out pretty quickly.

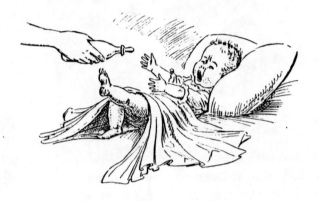

—Tricia Chandler

CORNS

Boil a potato in its skin. After it is nice and soft, take the skin off and put the inside of it next to the corn.

To get the full benefit of the peeling, it has to be left on for about twelve hours.

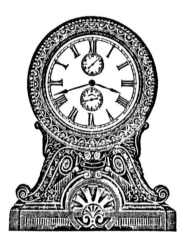

At the end of that time, the corn should feel much better.

—Kelly Murphy

COUGHS

My Grandmother, Vera Klostermann, uses the juice of a lemon, a teaspoon of honey, and a little water to help her cough.

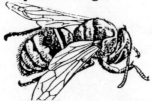

The mixture is heated. Then one teaspoon is taken every half hour.

—Travis Lahey

My grandmother, Mary Timmerman, from Dickeyville, Wisconsin, used this remedy for a cough. She told me it works very well, and figures it's just as good as a lot of medicine.

What she does is to take one cup of lard and one tablespoon of sugar. She mixes this together. 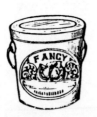 Then she browns the mixture in a skillet for five or six minutes. After this, she puts it in a regular-sized bowl and lets it set for about two hours.

This turns into a kind of a candy. But it isn't like most candy. What you'll be doing if you use this is sucking on something that tastes real bad!

—Stacy Timmerman

When my grandma was a little girl, she would often get a bad cough.

Grandma's family lived a long way from the nearest doctor, so her mother had to care for her as best she could all by herself.

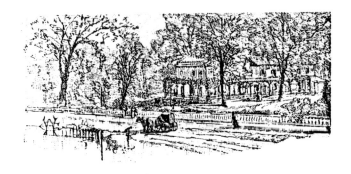

What her mother would do was to mix an ounce of glycerine along with two ounces of honey.

To this she would add a half ounce of lemon juice and mix it real well in a small container.

She'd give Grandma some of that mixture, and it worked real well. Grandma told me that soon after taking some of that stuff her mother would mix up for her, she'd get over her coughing.

—Mandy Allen

My grandma, Rose Goss, from Soldiers Grove told me when she was a little girl if she had a bad cough, her mother would give her some really gross stuff.

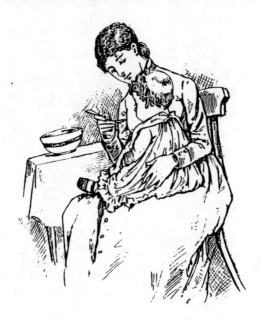

It was one half of a teaspoon of kerosene mixed with one-half teaspoon of sugar. My grandma had to drink it. I know if I had to drink that I'd get even sicker.

—Kathy Geasland

Stuffed up? Try breathing eucalyptus for about
ten minutes.

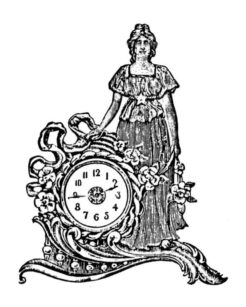

Just put some in water and boil the water so
somes team comes off real good.

The steam should open up your nasal passages
so you're not so congested.

It's like breathing a cough drop through your
nose.

—Sarah M. Young

(49)

COW ITCH

Back around the beginning of the 1890's a lot of children ran around with bare feet during the summer. Come the first warm day and most of the kids in town would shed their shoes, some of them not puttin' shoes back on until fall again.

It wouldn't be too long after the children started going barefooted that some of them would get what they called Cow Itch.

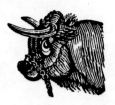

I don't know why they called it Cow Itch. It wasn't supposed to have anything to do with cows.

It did have to do with dryness of the skin and the skin between the toes cracking. Along with that went itching and burning.

Mary Harris' mother would tie a piece of wool yarn around the toes near the cracked skin.

Maybe it wasn't really a cure. Maybe it was just a reminder for the child to wear shoes.

—Amy Bader

(50)

CROUP

Hilda Chandler, who was born and raised in Platteville, used several home remedies with her children as they were growing up.

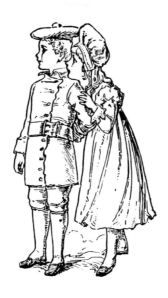

When any of her children had the croup, she would put a string of beads around their neck. She said the beads had to be put on so they were nice and snug. She thought that this helped keep the child's neck warm so that it would help them get over the croup.

—Tricia Chandler

REMEDIES FROM MY FATHER'S FAMILY

In my father's family, there was always some kerosene around the house since they used it in lamps, lanterns, and so forth.

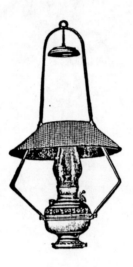

But that kerosene had another use besides being used in lamps and starting fires in the old cookstove.

That kerosene was also used to cure the croup.

Whoever had a case of the croup would simply breathe the vapors from a teaspoon of sugar in kerosene, and they were well on their way to being cured.

—Sarah Smidt

A CURE FOR THE CROUP

Great-Grandma Dorothy Tesch often developed a chest cold when she was a child.

She steamed sliced onions in lard or butter. Then she added tobacco to the hot steamed onions. This poultice was then put onto her chest.

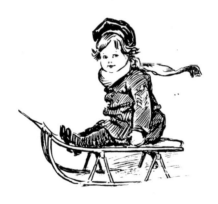

The mixture was left on for thirty minutes. Grandma Dorothy said that you could put the mixture directly on the chest, and flannel could be wrapped over the area. She warned to be careful that the mixture was not too hot for bare skin.

Grandma Dorothy said it worked for her family.

—Valerie Mumm

CUTS

Cure For A Cut

When Grandma Jenny was young, she cut her hand when she was playing. In order to get the infection out, her mother made a dressing called a poultice. The poultice consisted of a mixture of bread soaked in water.

Her mother would put it into a bag made out of gauze, and tape the bag on for as long as it took to get the infection out.

—Corey Jenny

When my Grandmother Rounds was a young girl, she got a bad cut on her foot. In her day, they didn't see a doctor often. So, to prevent infection in that foot her mother would heat a pan of water and put two handfuls of ashes in the water.

By soaking her foot in the water, it drew out any infections and made it heal quickly.

—Cory Pink

Remedy for a Deep Cut

My Grandfather told me about a home remedy that they used when he was a boy.

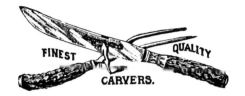

FINEST QUALITY

CARVERS.

This was for a person who had a deep cut.

The person treating the cut would clean it first and then spread unsalted lard on it to keep the wound clean and prevent infection. Then the cut would be wrapped in a bandage, and it would heal on its own. Grandpa knows this remedy worked because when he was a boy about my age he cut his finger right down to the bone.

His mother used the lard, bandaged the finger with a homemade splint, and it healed without a scar. Nowadays a cut like that would need stitches.

—Bryan Popp

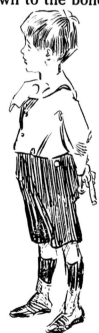

(55)

For a bad cut, an answer can be found out in the woods. All you have to do is to cut one of those dry puff balls open and squirt the powder that's inside right onto the cut. That will stop the bleeding.

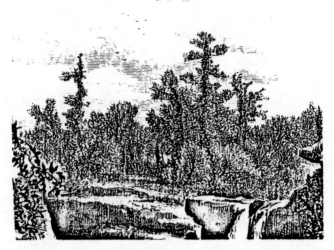

Since those puff balls are around only in the summer and early fall, it's best if you wait 'til then to get cut.

—Aaron Lange

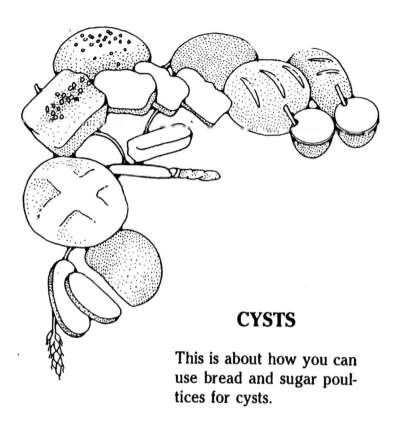

CYSTS

This is about how you can use bread and sugar poultices for cysts.

Grandma Sharon Jones got this old remedy from her mother, Dorothy Shanley, a long time ago.

She would take a piece of bread, put a sprinkle of sugar on it, then put some warm milk over the sugar. The bread was put right over the cyst and covered with gauze. It was left on there for two or three hours and repeated as necessary.

This acted as a drawing salve.

—Jennifer Uher

(57)

DIAPER RASH

Cornstarch was often used years ago as a means of controlling diaper rash.

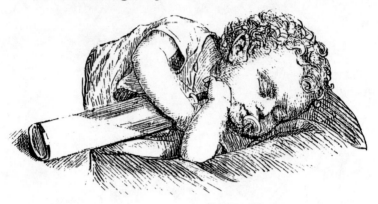

All the mother had to do was to sprinkle some of the starch into the baby's diaper, and things would go a lot better for the little fellow.

—Stacey Bast

Another good cure for diaper rash is to put some white flour in the oven until it turns brown. Sprinkle that in the diaper to both prevent and to cure diaper rash.

—Kathie Dreessens

DIARRHEA

I was told by my grandma that if you get some sort of disease that ends up giving you diarrhea, there is a cure for you waiting right out in the woods. That's blackberry juice. All you have to do is to drink some blackberry juice.

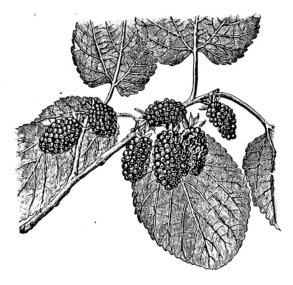

Some folks do that and don't even have diarrhea.

—Tiffany Klosterman

HOW TO DIET

Grandma Annabelle Weier told me a story of how her family lost weight back when she was a kid.

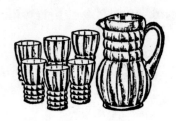

If someone was a bit chubby, they would swallow a tapeworm.

My grandma's aunt, Catherine McKernen was the first one in our family to try this. She swallowed a tape worm with some bread, and washed it down with some iced tea. She said that she hardly knew it was in her.

After about five months, the tape worm had done its job by eating all the food inside of Catherine's stomach.

She then swallowed castor oil. It was supposed to kill the worm.

At first she wasn't quite sure if she had killed it. She finally figured she had, though, since she gained five pounds in only a week.

—Lindsay Weier

DROPSY

Just a few weeks ago, I got a letter from my Grandma Marcella Schaefer telling me about what her mother had told her.

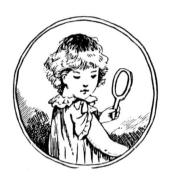

She told that when she was a youngster she had scarlet fever. While she was recovering, she developed dropsy and her grandmother used to heat bran bags and pack them around her to make her sweat.

She was also given herb tea. This acted as a diaretic and helped to get rid of the fluid.

The treatment must have been a success because Grandma's mother lived to be ninety-three years old.

—Tiffany Klosterman

EARACHES

This remedy is for earaches.

When my Grandma Ruth Allen got an earache, her mother took a cotton ball and put pepper on it.

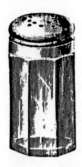

When she took the cotton ball out later, the earache was gone.

—Matt Allen

When my Great-Grandpa Round's children were small and would get an earache, they would heat up a hickory stick until the sap would run out. Then they would put drops of the sap into the ear to keep it from hurting.

—Cory Pink

My Great-Grandma Ruby Barto was a little girl in the late 1800's. Back then, people had a strange cure for earaches.

When an earache got so bad that a person couldn't stand it, someone who smoked would blow a huge puff of smoke into the aching ear. This would make it feel better right away. You can just imagine how unsanitary that was.

—Mahrya Draheim

My Great-Grandmother Ethel Butson tells of a home remedy that she remembered from when she was a little girl.

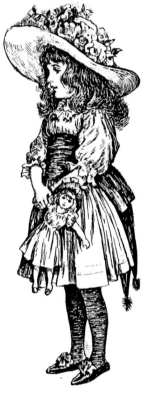

She didn't have this done to herself, but a friend of hers did when they were just children.

When this friend of Great-Grandmother's would get an earache, her father would make her sleep through the night with a warm raisin stuck in each ear. It was just like the ear plugs you can put in your ears when you go swimming, except they were warm raisins.

Great-grandmother told that her friend would get relief from the pain right away and wake up in the morning with the earache totally gone.

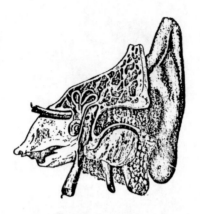

While it did make Great-grandmother's friend's earache feel better, it might have not been a real good idea because that person is hard of hearing now. Maybe one of those raisins did that to her.

—Ryan Leibfried

A story from Potosi, Wisconsin, tells much the same about using smoke for an earache, but the smoke had to be from a man's pipe.

—Damian Eveland

Another good cure for earaches is to lay a nice warm cat on the side of the person's head.

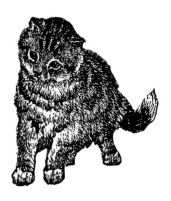

And, then, of course, what you could do if the CAT had an earache, too, is to lay the cat so its ear was right next to . . . . No, I don't think that would work.

—Stacey Bast

When my Grandma Chandler of Arthur, Wisconsin, was younger, back in the 1930's, she ran into an interesting home remedy.

The remedy was for earache in a newborn baby.

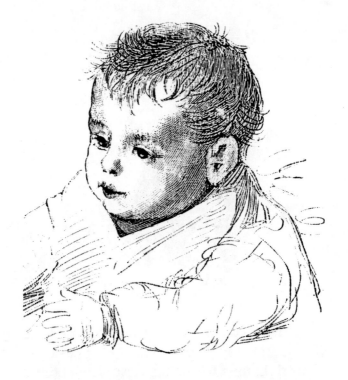

If a newborn baby came down with an earache, it was common practice to put some mother's milk in the aching ear. It was supposed to help cure the earache and quiet the baby down.

—Pat Chandler

Yet another remedy for an earache was to put some sweet oil in the ear.

It was necessary to let the oil "work" in there for about ten minutes. Then you had to drain out the remaining oil.

—Mitchell Harrison

If folks were out of sweet oil, they would often use the old sliced onion remedy for an earache.

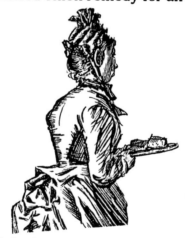

What you'd do for that one was to fry up half an onion. You would then put it in a cloth so it wouldn't burn the person and hold it up against the ear for anywhere from three to ten minutes.

—Mitchell Harrison

My Aunt Lila from Platteville not only told me about this remedy, but proved it worked by using it on my cousin. And it worked well for him.

This is a remedy for earaches.

What she would do was to boil up some sesame oil with a clove of garlic in it.

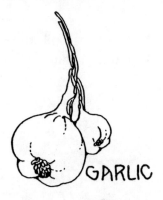

GARLIC

After that oil had cooked up a while with the garlic, she would strain it and put it into a little jar.

Whenever anyone got an earache, Aunt Lila would get some of that oil out and put it into the ear.

She found it would work just the way it was, but would work better if it was warmed up first.

—Ashlesha Sharma

ECZEMA

Another one of Grandpa's home remedies was what could be used when he was troubled with eczema.

He would make a lotion of one tablespoon of fresh rendered unsalted lard and one tablespoon of yellow powdered suphur.

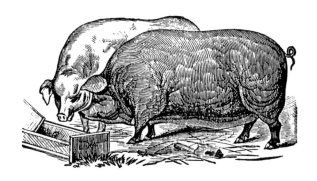

The lard and the sulphur were mixed well together and rubbed onto the skin to clear it up.

—Stacey Bast

FEVER

One of my favorite home remedies is the one that my great-great grandmother used on my Great-Uncle Donald.

A doctor had been at the house to take care of Donald, but he didn't have any medicine that would break the terrible fever that Uncle Donald had.

The doctor told the family that they best simply make Donald as comfortable as they could 'cause he probably wasn't going to last the night.

Great-Great Grandma just started frying onions. After she had a batch ready, she'd put them in a large square of two pieces of flannel sewn together to make sort of a pocket. Then she put this on his chest.

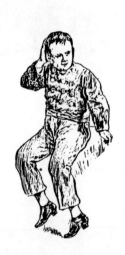

Within a couple of hours, the fever was broken and Uncle Donald recovered real fast after that.

—Denise Wetter

One winter when my dad was little, he got a real bad fever. His temperature got up to 103°. So my grandma took a blanket and spread snow all over it.

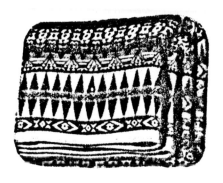

Then she wrapped him up in it to take the temperature down.

—Benji Fowler

FRECKLES

If you get freckles and you don't want them, you can wash your face in buttermilk to get rid of them.

—Brent Mann

Another cure for freckles comes to us from my grandmother, Millie Roddick.

Grandmother Roddick had a lot of freckles when she was a little girl. They way she tells it, she must have done a lot of complaining about her freckles.

"My brother pulled what I thought at the time was an awfully mean trick.

"We were out in the pasture where there were some cows, and of course, there were lots of cow pies, too.

"I guess I didn't know how tired my brother was about my constant complaining about my freckles.

"And I don't know if he really knew anything about the effects of cow manure on freckles or not. But what he did was to deliberately trip me so I fell right smack into one of those terrible cow pies.

"I suppose most people know how mad a girl can get at her brother anyway. Well, I was just plenty mad at him for that trick. I landed right in that thing face first, and got it all over me."

"My brother, of course, just took off running, leaving me in that terrible state."

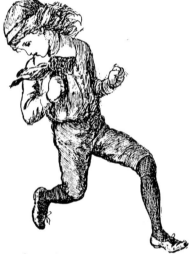

"By the time I got back to the house, that manure that I couldn't wipe off had dried and hardened."

"Believe me, I cried all the way home."

"When I got to the house, my mother worked on scrapping and washing that off my face. She noticed that wherever that manure had been, the freckles were gone.

"So, my brother actually did me a real favor that day."

—Jeremy Reuter

FROST BITE

How To Warm Frost-Bitten Hands.

I talked to my grandmother, Annabelle Weier. She told me that every morning she and her brothers and sisters would walk to school.

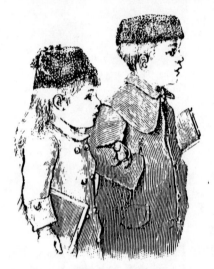

In the winter, she said her hands would be terribly cold.

When they got to school, her teacher would have her put them in cold water. She told me the water warmed them up nicely. For some reason, it would seem to warm them up faster than if she put them in warm water.

—Lindsay Weier

GALLSTONES

My great-great-great-grandma used to take a tablespoon of olive oil every day to soften her gallstones.

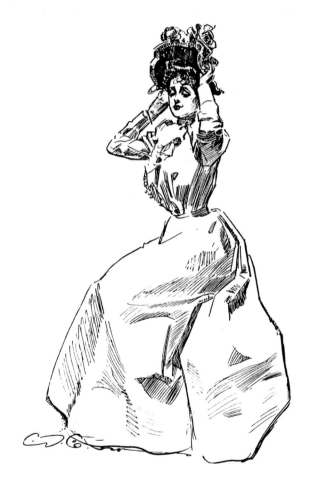

—Stacey Bast

(75)

GANGRENE

A Cow Manure Cure

During World War I, soldiers would get gangrene in wounds that hadn't been taken care of properly. If that happened, they would have to get the part with gangrene cut off. If they didn't do that, they could easily die.

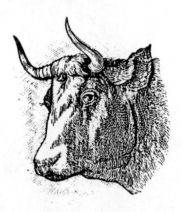

My great-grandmother said that cow manure was put in the soldier's boots until the infection was gone. She found out from the doctor later that it worked because the bacteria in the manure were stronger than the bacteria in the gangrene. He figured the manure bacteria would kill the others.

Who would have ever thought that cow manure could save a person's life?

—Bethany Kies

HANGNAILS

Hangnails are pieces of skin hanging loose near the side or root of a fingernail.

Very often a piece of skin breaking loose that way will get infected and very sore.

Curing a hangnail in the old days simply involved breaking open an egg and removing that thin moist lining that is just on the inside of the shell.

It's kind of a slimy thin thing that separates the egg shell from the egg inside.

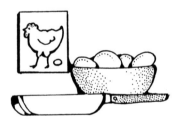

You simply apply this moist lining inside of the shell directly onto the hangnail.

It is important that you let it dry and harden. Once the lining is good and dry you can peel it off the finger and the hangnail will be gone. It will be cured.

—Cory Burgess

HICCUPS

When my grandmother, Lillian White, was a little girl and had the hiccups, she was really unhappy about it. She tried every thing she could possibly think of to get rid of those hiccups.

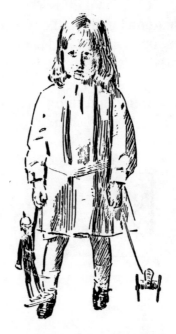

Mrs. White had an answer, though, and it worked real well.

She plugged Lillian's nose and covered her mouth for almost half a minute.

That did the job every time. Lillian got over those hiccups right away.

—Kelly Thomas

HIVES

When my mother, Joanie Gassman, was a little girl, she'd eat too many strawberries and break out in hives. Every time that happened, her mother would have to come up with a home remedy that cured the itching right away.

She'd mix up some baking soda and water to make a paste that she'd put on the hives.

My mother didn't like that treatment, but it worked.

—Rhonda Gassman

INDIGESTION

Carmen Aspromonte tells about a home remedy that had been used in her family for indigestion.

They would boil a cup of water and add several bay leaves. They would then remove the bay leaves and add one teaspoon of sugar.

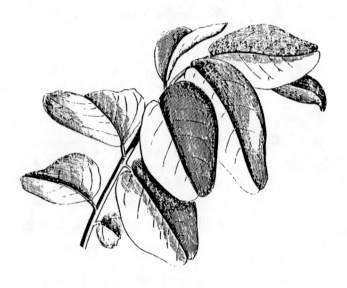

The bay leaf tea would immediately alkalize the acid condition which caused the indigestion.

—Daniel MacKenzie

INFECTIONS

A "Cow Pie" Remedy

I heard this story from my grandmother who lived on a farm here in Wisconsin.

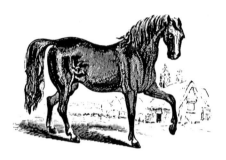

Her father used this to cure a horse's foot infection.

When a horse had an infection, her father would put some warm cow manure in a bag. Then he would put the horse's foot in the bag and tie the top of it around the critter's leg.

This warm cow pie drew the infection out of the leg. My grandma said this remedy worked real well.

I don't have a horse, but if I did have one and it turned up lame from an infection, I think I'd take him to a vet instead.

—Damian Eveland

This remedy for infections was used by my great grandmother who lived in Bell Center, Wisconsin, back in the 1930's.

It was a simple remedy made only of bread and milk.

Great-Grandmother would soak the bread in the milk so it was good and soggy.

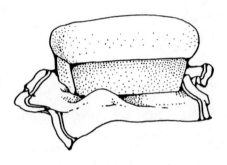

She'd put that really, really wet bread right on the spot that was infected, and then put a bandage over it so it would not get rubbed off in the night as the person slept.

Come morning the infection would be all cleared up.

—Stephanie Jones

My grandmother from Benton, Wisconsin, told me about when she was ten years old in 1937 and she was roller skating by her house and fell down.

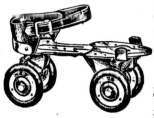

She ended up with pieces of gravel in her hand, giving her a deep infection.

So my great-grandmother soaked some bread in milk and wrapped it around my grandmother's hand. After a while, the poultice drew the infection to the surface. This is supposed to work by the milk activating the yeast in the bread, which then draws out the infection.

—Troy Swift

Another bread and milk poultice comes to us from Judy Moriarty. When Judy was a young girl her mother would treat her daughter's infections with bread and milk also.

This remedy, however, calls for the milk to be well heated before the bread is put into it.

It also called for repeated applications if it didn't work the first time.

—Carrie Moriarty

When my great-great-grandpa would get an infected finger, he'd go out into the woods and find a plantain weed.

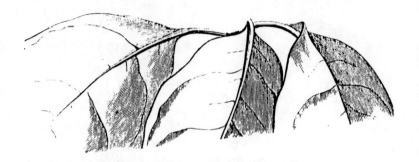

He'd bring some leaves back to the house where he'd wash and dry them well.

He'd crush the leaves with the flat part of a knife and then wrap the things around the infected finger just like it was some kind of bandage.

Finally, he'd put a regular bandage over the plantain weed leaves.

Within a short time, the infection would be drawn out of the finger and it would heal right away.

—Stacey Bast

LARYNGITIS

My great-great-aunt Verna tells about how they used to cure laryngitis in their family with a few drops of kerosene mixed in with some lard.

This mixture would be rubbed well on the neck. Then they would wrap the neck good to keep that stuff working well.

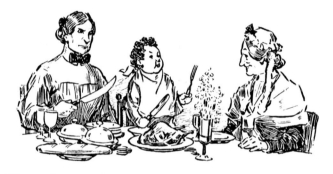

Then, just to be sure they got that neck good and greased up, they would have the patient eat a lot of bread dipped in cooking grease.

—Tonya Nall

LICE

My Great-Aunt Marie Parkenson tells of some interesting home remedies from when she was a young girl.

Marie lived with her family on a farm near Darlington, and the family had many occasions to doctor themselves there on the farm.

If someone in the family was unlucky enough to have head lice, Marie's mother would go to the shed and get a mug of kerosene.

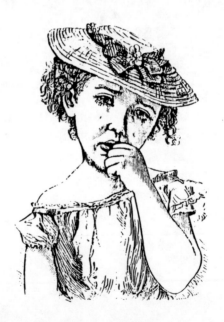

She'd dip a rag in the kerosene and thoroughly rub the head until it was soaked good and wet.

This procedure was repeated about a half hour later.

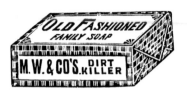

Then a regular bar of soap was used to wash out the kerosene.

No side effects were ever noticed that she could remember except that the kid would smell like an old kerosene lamp for a couple of days.

One thing that Aunt Marie would do was to be sure the kid didn't get too near the stove if it was going.

—Aaron Bartels

MEASLES

I was told by my Grandmother Virginia Sanches that when you have the measles you should rub lemon juice on your body.

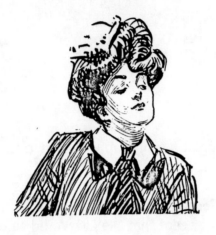

—Tiffany Klosterman

A tea made from hops leaves was given to help children break out with measles.

—Heather Butson

MORNING SICKNESS

My mother, Janel Wunderlin, was pregnant when her grandmother, Doris McCabe, told her about a remedy for morning sickness.

Not only did Great-Grandmother McCabe tell my mother about the cure, but she fixed some up for her.

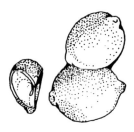

All it amounted to was to get some water good and hot, then add a few squirts of lemon juice to the water.

Great-Grandmother let the mixture of water and lemon juice cool just enough so that my mother could drink it.

In a very short time, Mother was feeling a lot better and was convinced it was due to that remedy her grandmother fixed for her.

I kind of wonder how that tastes, but don't think I'll mess with it until I think I might need it.

—Jenny Wunderlin

MUMPS

This remedy for mumps comes from Leone Hensel.

Put wet rags on the patient's cheeks and put a warm wool cloth around the throat.

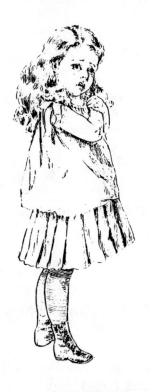

—Kim Roskom

NETTLES

When my dad was a kid, he would go out into the woods a lot. And when he came home, he usually had a lot of good old fashioned nettle stings.

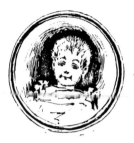

My grandmother would always put caladril on those stings. One day, though, she was out of caladril and told my dad to get on down to the creek and put creek mud on it.

That seemed to work just as well as the medicine she usually used.

—Corey Jenny

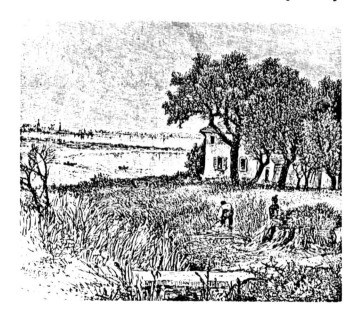

NOSEBLEEDS

One day a friend of mine got a nose bleed, and it bled and bled. It simply would not stop.

When his mother found out what was happening, she used an old family remedy.

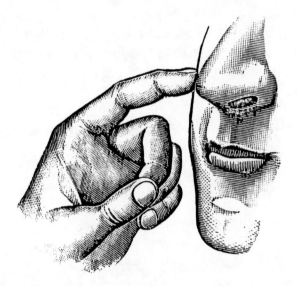

She rolled a piece of brown paperbag up into a tight roll and pressed it up inside against his upper lip. Within a couple of minutes, the bleeding stopped.

—Jodi Lynch

POISONS

My Great-Great, Aunt Verna grew up near Sauk City, Wisconsin, and recalls some of the remedies they used when she was a child.

She remembers how Black Jack wagon axle grease was used as a medicine! Her family believed that that particular wagon axle grease would pull blood poisons out of either humans or animals.

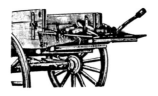

I just can't imagine eating that stuff.

—Tonya Nall

POISON IVY

One day many years ago my Grandma Lenore Anderson and her friend were out picking red raspberries to have her mother make some of her prize raspberry jam.

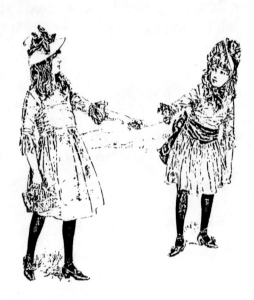

Before the day was over, both girls really wished that they had never heard of picking raspberries, 'cause they got into some poison ivy out there.

A family friend came to visit and noticed Grandma Anderson's scratching. He asked what the problem was and she told of how she had gotten into that poison ivy. The visitor went down by the creek in search of some Jack-In-The-Box. Finding some, he took it back to the house and spread some juice from the stem on the affected area. Within a short time, the effects of the poison ivy was gone.

—John Diedrichs

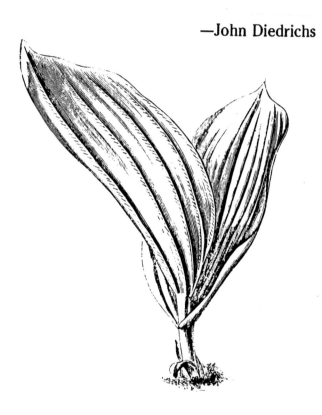

A good cure for posion ivy is to break a milk weed stem and smear that thick white juice onto the area.

—Stephen Buchs

(95)

PREMATURE BABIES

This home remedy is one that was done by a doctor, but it was still done there at the family's home, using what they had to do with.

It all happened in 1926 when my father's twin brothers, Louis and Levi Richardson, were born.

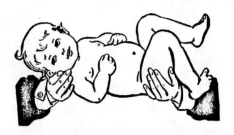

The boys were premature and came as quite a shock to their mother who was only a seventeen-year-old at the time.

The Richardsons lived in a little cabin down along the Grant River near Potosi, Wisconsin. But they got a doctor there when they realized that my grandmother was going to have her baby and have it way early.

Well, that "baby" turned out to be two of them and tiny as they could be.

The doctor knew right away that the babies needed to be in some kind of incubator but had nothing of that sort with him, of course.

So, that's where my grandma's cookstove there in the kitchen came in.

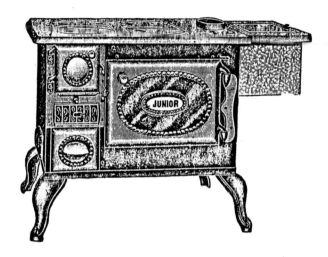

The doctor told what he wanted to do so the family scurried around and got that cookstove going on real low heat.

Leaving the door open, the doctor put those two little premature babies right there in the oven of that stove!

That doctor sure knew what he was doing because he not only saved those two little babies, but they thrived and grew.

When Louis and Levi grew up, they both got to be well over six feet tall and became farmers.

—Jill Richardson

PREVENTIONS

My grandma told me that a little bag of asofinity worn around the neck would ward off disease. It's so smelly it would keep everyone around you away, too. Besides that, it's hard to spell.

—Tiffany Klosterman

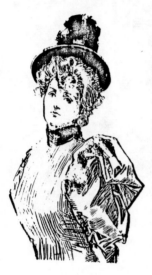

Marie Roberts of Stevens Point, Wisconsin, has a remedy she still takes in order to stay healthy. Every day she puts some crushed lobelia seeds mixed with vinegar in a glass, a teaspoonful of cayenne pepper or crushed garlic loves. Then she drinks this concoction. These must work because she just never gets sick.

—Katie Wroblewski

PUNCTURES

I can remember my grandpa, William Hauser, telling me about when he was a kid and would step on a nail. He said that his mother made him step in a fresh cow pie two or three times. He didn't care for that treatment, but it did heal him up at that.

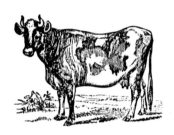

—Nick Hauser

My mother tells about a remedy she recalls from her childhood.

She would often get a puncture on her foot from a weed stalk or running through a hay field barefooted.

When she did that, she would limp over to the side of the field and find a milkweed plant. She'd rub the white, milky fluid from the stem onto her wound to stop the bleeding.

—Amanda Kitto

(99)

My grandmother, Maude Fitzgerald, told me one day that her mother was working in the kitchen and heard her son crying.

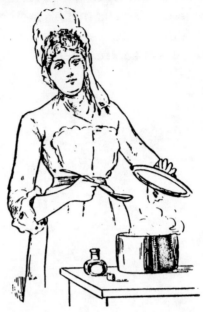

"Mother!! Help! Help! I got something in my foot!"

My great-grandma ran outside to see to Eddy, her son.

"Oh, my!" she exclaimed. "You've stepped on a rusty nail!"

She yelled to my grandma, "Maude, go get your father!"

"Tell your mother not to worry," Great-Grandpa said. "I've got a remedy that my daddy taught me that'll fix him right up!"

(100)

Great-Grandpa then ran out into the pasture and got a fresh warm cow flop, scooped it into a bucket and brought it to Eddy. Then he made Eddy put his foot into that bucket for about fifteen minutes.

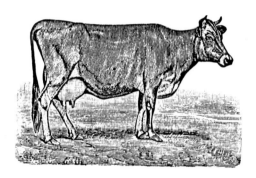

Grandma Maude explained that she figured that her father believed the strong aroma of the cow flop would draw the poison right out of Eddy's foot.

But, I know if I stepped on a rusty nail, I'd rather go to the doctor. His office would probably smell better!

—Kelli Kruser

PUPPIES THAT WHINE

When our family first got our puppy, it whined all the time for the first day.

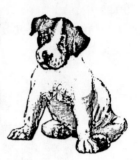

I called my grandma to tell her how sad the poor little critter sounded.

She said to put a hot water bottle wrapped in a towel in with the puppy as well as a ticking clock. She told me that the puppy would think

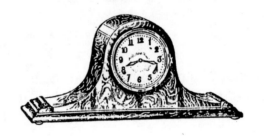

the warm bottle was its mother, and the ticking of the clock would remind it of his mother's heartbeat.

So, that's what we did, and it worked!

—Shannon Van Natta

QUINSY

My great grandmother used to have to take lots of gross home remedies from her grandmother.

One of these was for what they called quinsy which was a condition of swollen glands in the throat.

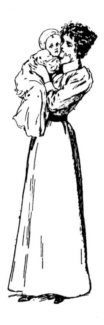

What her grandmother would do was to cook up some potatoes with the skin and dirt still on them. She'd mash them and wrap them in a poultice for the neck. That was supposed to move the pain down into the chest where the doctor could get to it.

—Matt MacKenzie

(103)

RINGWORM

Hazel Cline tells about a cure for the skin disease of ringworm that is supposed to be a very old home remedy.

The husk of a black walnut is broken open and rubbed on the ring-shaped patches that give this disease its name.

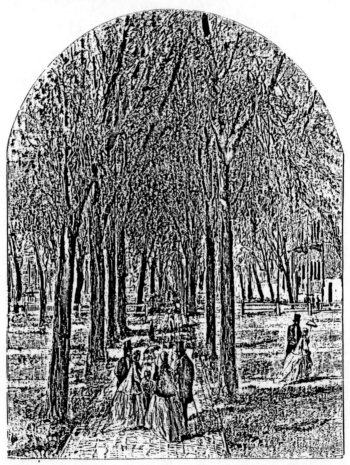

The disease is supposed to be cured in a very short time if this is used.

This cure works best if the husk is damp, so that some of the juices get onto the ringworm area. So this cure works better in the summer and fall when the husk is still moist.

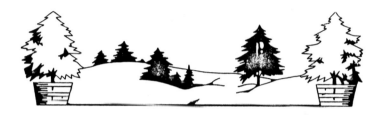

In the winter, of course, the walnut husks are all dried up. Maybe a person could use one of those dried-up husks if he wet it down first.

—Amy Chase

SINUS PROBLEMS

My grandma makes chicken noodle soup once in awhile. But, its's different from most ordinary chicken soups.

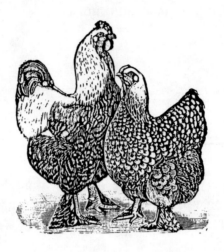

The recipe calls for lots and lots of spice. So, anytime we have any sinus problems, we just ask grandma for some of her special chicken noodle soup.

And, it sure tastes better 'n most stuff that comes out of little bottles or in pills.

—Quintin Stoltz

SKUNK SMELL

Argued with a skunk lately? If so, you don't need to move out of your house just because of the smell. You can solve the problem just by taking a bath in tomato juice. It really takes away the smell.

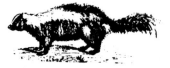

—Sarah M. Young

One day late in the summer many years ago my Frandmother Gladys and her little brother Walter were walking in their woods in back of their parents' farm.

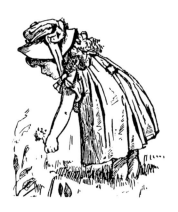

As they got near the middle of the woods, they remembered having been told to stay away from the creek because "unpredictable" animals roamed the area.

Walter and Gladys were having way too much fun to pay much attention to such silly rules so they went in there anyway. After all, the water was so clear and crisp and really, really fun to play in.

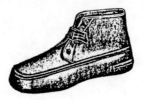

They took off their shoes, played in the water, and skipped rocks.

Time slipped away quickly and the pair soon found it was time to go in order to get home in time for chores, even though both of them were still wet.

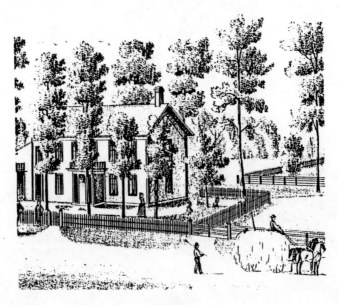

On the way back to the house, Walter accidentally tripped over a stone, scraped his knee and found himself face to face with a real problem, a very upset skunk.

Those two might have gotten away with the whole situation except for one thing. Gladys decided she needed to do a bunch of screaming about that woodland kitty.

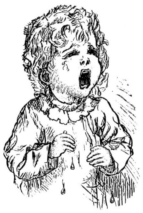

That's all it took. Gladys raised so much racket that the skunk got scared and sprayed them both.

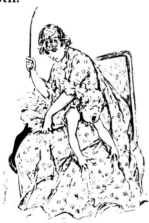

Even the spanking the two of them expected when they got home didn't slow the pair down any as they tried to put as much distance between them and the skunk as they could.

When Walter and Gladys finally got back to the house, their parents were so busy trying to get past that terrible smell they plumb forgot to dole out any punishment.

They ended up burying their children up to their necks in a dirt pile so the dirt would absorb that skunk odor.

Walter and Gladys both got the good old goose grease and turpentine to cure the sniffles they both developed from wading around in that cold water.

Walter got an extra treatment of warm milk and bread to heal the cuts and scrapes he got from the fall that led to the skunk incident.

—Andrea Honshel

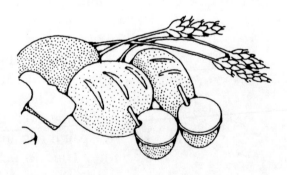

SLEEPING PROBLEMS

If you want to go to sleep in a hurry, just follow these directions:

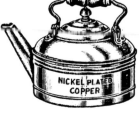

Take one cup of milk and one teaspoon of honey. Heat the mixture until it's fairly hot. Then get into bed and drink the potion slowly.

—David Charles

This remedy is one that comes from my grandma.

When a child couldn't fall asleep, mothers would put "Yerba Luisa" leaves under the child's pillow. After lying down for a while, the child would become sleepy.

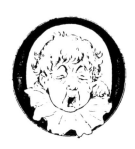

Another use for the Yerba Luisa leaves was for the easing of pain in the stomach. It would be boiled and then served as a tea.

Also, the leaves make a very pretty house plant.

—Jenny Lolita McFall

SLIVERS

One day my grandma got a sliver when she was just a child. Her mother bought some LEKSELL which is a Tootsie Roll looking kind of stuff made in Sweden.

They melted that strange-looking stuff on the blade of a kitchen knife and then smeared it on the sliver. It sort of hardened up like wax from a candle would and they left it on overnight.

The next morning Grandma's mother peeled that LEKSELL off, and it pulled that sliver off with it.

—Meredith Lee

SNAKE BITES

For snake bites, my great grandma had a sure-fire cure.

She'd take a live chicken and cut it in half and put half of the chicken on the bite.

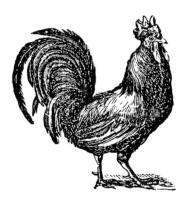

The chicken turned black as it drew the poison out. They would keep repeating this until the chicken would no longer turn black. Sometimes they would have to use two or three chickens.

Snake bites weren't so hard on folks in the community after they started using the little trick. 'Course, it was kind of tough on chickens.

—Sarah McCabe

SNAKEBITE REMEDY

When the American Indians got bitten by a snake, they had a remedy they often used.

It involved digging up snakeroot. Snakeroot is the root of any of a number of different kinds of plants, all of which were supposed to cure snakebite.

Some of the particular plants were the Virginia snakeroot, Button snakeroot, White snakeroot, and the Bugbane plant.

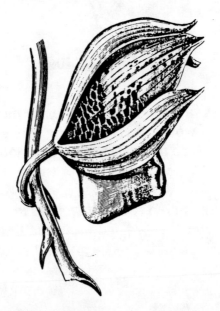

They would grind the root up into a granular like powder. That would then be put right on the bite and left there for about four hours.

The Indians had the idea that the powder from the roots of certain plants had the power to cure a snakebite.

They thought it worked by drawing the poison right out of the bite.

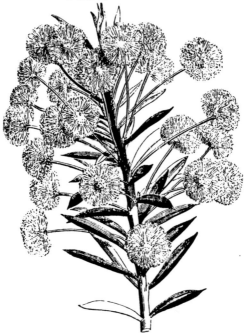

Since it could take a long time to find the right plants and to grind up the roots, the Indians would try to keep some of the ground-up roots on hand. That way, they could use it right away if anyone got bit by a snake.

—Brooke Palmer

SNAKE BITE IN CATTLE

This remedy come from a book of old remedies that my Grandma Georgia Halverson has kept for many years.

Grandma Halverson says that she had lots of those remedies used on her by her mother.

She laughed and said that this one never had been used on her 'cause she never did get bitten by a snake.

"Besides that, this one's for cows, not people."

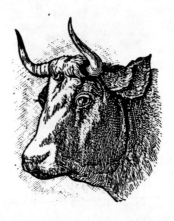

Cattle or horses are usually bitten in the feet. When this is the case, all that is needed is to drive the animal into a mudhole and keep it there for a few hours.

Grandma said that the mud will pull the poison right out of the bite.

If they are bitten on the nose, then you have to tie the mud on the bite in such a way that you don't cut off their air.

Grandma said that if she had to live in a place where there were a bunch of snakes, she wouldn't live there unless there was a creek nearby.

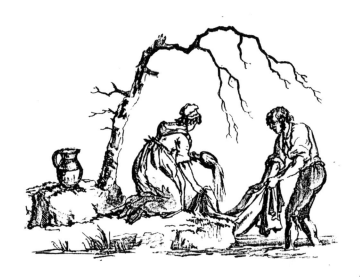

—Kelly Murphy

SORES

A neighbor of mine, Gladys Anderson, has a bunch of remedies for this and that. She told me a number of things that you can do for a sore, for example.

She explained that you can use salt, goose goop, a sheep hide, white sugar, or sheep tallow.

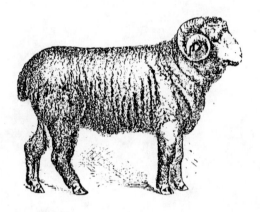

If you want to treat a sore with salt, you just dissolve it in water and let it flow across the sore. The salt will draw out the infection.

You can made a cure for sores with goose goop. You simply cook the fat, and work it into the sore while it is still warm.

The sheep hide is the easiest of all to use. What you do is to sleep on the hide all night.

It works well to cover a sore with white sugar or to rub sheep tallow on it like a salve.

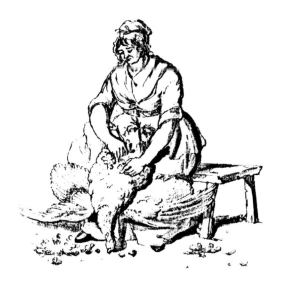

—Mitchell Harrison

Occasionally my ancestors used a poultice made of some of Grandpa's chewed tobacco. It was disgusting, but a sure cure for any sore.

—Tonya Nall

SPRAINS

According to the old timers in my family, if you ever sprained your wrist or ankle, you could cure it by wrapping a wet brown paper bag around it.

—Brent Mann

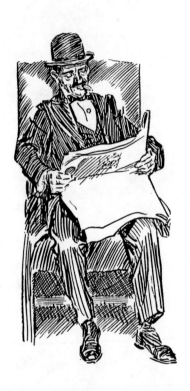

STINGS

My grandmother from Benton, Wisconsin, used to make a remedy of baking soda and water. This paste was used to take the pain out of the bites or stings of wasps, bees, hornets, and ants.

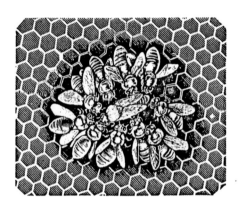

She'd just quickly mix up that paste and slap it right onto the bite or sting before it had time to swell up the skin.

Before long the pain would be gone.

—Troy Swift

My grandmother's friend, Mrs. Rosemary Chance, told me about a really good home remedy for bee stings.

In their home, if somebody was stung by a bee, they would use calamine lotion on it. Mrs. Chance said that the calamine lotion would work right away so the sting would stop hurting almost as soon as they put the lotion on.

She also told me that another thing they would use if they didn't have any calamine lotion was simple mud.

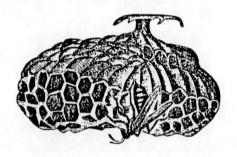

The mud remedy would work if they were down by the creek or out in the woods where it would be a long way back to the house to get some calamine lotion.

Another thing they would do would be to quickly slice up an onion and then slap that fresh cut onion slice onto the area of the sting.

—Carriel Abing

STOMACH ACHES

A Sweet Peppermint Remedy

My grandmother had a sweet remedy for tummy aches. Her mother, Lorraine Drury, used to give my grandmother a drink consisting of hot water, oil of peppermint and sugar. Grandmother liked that so much that she used to pretend that she had a stomach ache just to get some.

—Lindsay Heiser

When my Grandma Maedean O'Conner came to visit, she told me about a home remedy she remembered from her childhood. It was catnip tea. This was used for upset stomachs or fussiness in babies and small children.

Grandma used to have to go out into the pasture and find catnip plants for her mother. It's a plant that grows wild and looks something like a thistle. But it was easy to tell it from a thistle because it had a smell all its own.

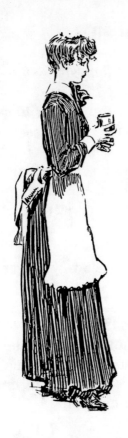

When my mother or her brother or sisters would be feeling bad, Grandma would steep some of that catnip like it was tea.

For wintertime use, Grandma would just dry some of those leaves and they would work just as well.

—Andy Placko

Vinegar Fizz

My grandma told me that when she had a tummy ache she would mix some baking soda and vinegar in a glass of water.

Just as it started to fizz and bubble, she'd drink it.

She said it tasted pretty badly the first time she tried it, but she got used to it and always felt better the next day.

—Kiley Goke

You know how Jello starts out as a powder, and your mother mixes it with warm water to make a sticky yucky mess that will then stiffen up to make good-tasting Jello?

Well, a good cure for an upset stomach is to drink a glass of the warm Jello before it stiffens up and while it is still good and warm.

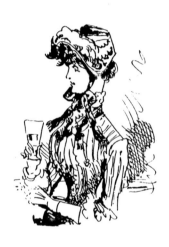

It's supposed to work by putting a coating on the inside of your stomach and calming it down.

—Shannon Jones

SUNBURN

A good cure for sunburn is a mixture of powdered soda and water.

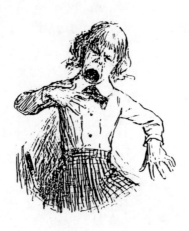

You have to be real careful when you put the mixture on so it doesn't hurt a lot. It helps if the mixture is very thin instead of pasty.

—Stephen Buchs

TARNISHED SILVER

This one isn't really a remedy for an illness that people get. I guess you could call tarnish on silver an illness that silver can get.

Anyway, here's a way to clean the tarnish off silver without going to a whole lot of work.

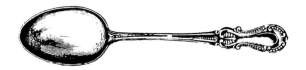

Line your sink with aluminum foil and put warm water with Tide in the sink. One cup of tide is plenty enough.

The silver should soak in that for a few minutes until all the tarnish is gone.

It doesn't do any better job than working real hard polishing it up, but it's a lot easier.

—Christy Moyer

THROAT THAT'S SORE

I got this remedy from my mother, Ann Gardner.

When she was a child and they didn't have any medicine in the house, they used this homemade medicine.

It was for sore throats and all they did was to mix warm water and salt. Mother said they usually used just a teaspoon in an average-sized glass of water.

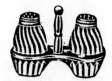 I had to try this once, and it was just awful.

Another remedy that my mother remembered was also for sore throats. It tastes a whole lot better and is regular tea but with a lot of honey added to it.

—Chris Gardner

This remedy for a sore throat has been passed down to me my Aunt Sue.

It started with my Grandpa Park who might have learned it from earlier members of the family.

All you have to do is to mix lemon juice and honey together.

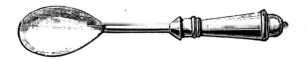

You're supposed to drink it warm, so it works well to heat the lemon juice up before you add the honey. That makes it mix better.

When the mixture is just about the right temperature, you drink it down and go to bed. The honey makes it stick to your throat, and the lemon juice makes it feel good.

—Amanda McFall

One kind of strange remedy for a sore throat is to put a wet rag on the throat and a dry rag on the face. No one is real sure exactly why this is supposed to work.

—Kim Roskom

I got this from my grandmother who lives in Potosi.

She remembered from when she was a little girl what her parents did for sore throats.

When Grandma had a sore throat her mother would cook up a goose and collect the fat that came off it.

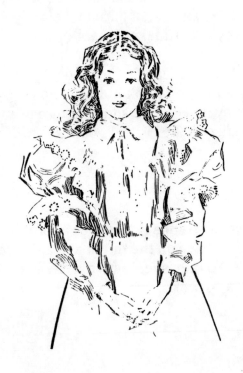

Great-Grandma would then let that fat cool down to a greasy mess and rub it real well onto Grandma's neck. Then Great-Grandma would tie a sock around Grandma's neck to keep that grease on there and keep it warm.

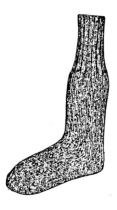

I guess it'd work, but it sure seems kind of gross to me.

—Damian Eveland

Got a Sore Throat?

This is a remedy that will truly knock your socks off!

Years ago people would wear their socks for about a week before changing them. You can just imagine how icky those socks would get between washings. Things can get kind of messy on the farm and you know the kinds of things that socks got walked in.

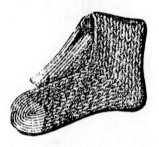

My great grandmother, Irene Kies, remembers when my grandpa and the rest of her children got sore throats.

Back in those days the doctor was too far away to come for just every little thing so our family had to do their own doctoring. 'Sides that, they often didn't have enough money for a doctor.

So Great-Grandma would take a dirty sock and wrap it around the sick child's throat. Before too long that sore throat would be gone and the kid could go back to school or out to play.

Great-Grandma isn't real sure just how that dirty sock remedy worked, but it did.

All I know is that I'm glad I don't have to do that nowadays. My friends would really laugh at me if I wore a dirty sock around my neck to school. I wouldn't even be what you'd call real excited about wearing 'em on my feet.

—Bethany Kies

My grandma's grandma told about a remedy for sore throats.

She said that what they used to do if someone in the family had a sore throat was to treat it with goose grease.

What they'd do was to find a dead goose and squeeze the lard out of it. Then they'd put it on a rag or towel.

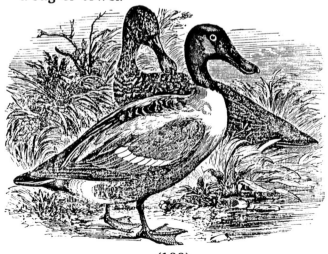

(133)

Then they'd lay that rag on the sick person's chest. The patient would feel better in three or four days.

I'm not real sure where a person goes to find a dead goose. I've never seen one.

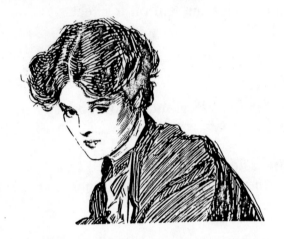

My mother told me that maybe you were supposed to cook the lard out of the goose instead of squeezing it out, but I'm just telling you what I know.

—Kiley Goke

Here's another "dead sock" cure. This is a remedy for a sore throat that my grandfather told me about.

The person with the sore throat was supposed to take the sock off his left foot and wrap it snugly around his neck.

(134)

And the foot of the sock has to be placed right over the person's throat.

Grandpa said that the remedy works best when the sock has been worn for several days before it gets used to cure the throat that way.

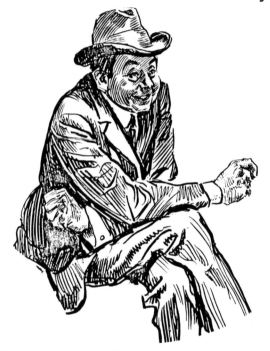

If it was up to me, I'd just as soon go ahead and have the sore throat.

—Bryan Popp

Years ago Kumar Chettiar woke up with a terrible sore throat. It was one of those sore throats so bad that he couldn't even swallow.

Kumar's mother, Seetha, looked into Kumar's throat and realized that he really had a bad one, and it was going to take a whole lot more than a little honey and whiskey to fix it up.

So Seetha brought out the big pans and fell back on an old family remedy that had been in the family a lot longer than anyone could remember.

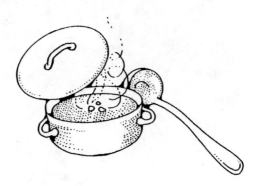

She mixed up four tablespoons of black pepper (whole), one tablespoon of coriander seed, and one teaspoon of cumin seed. She heated these altogether, dry, in a hot pan, then dumped them out and ground them into a fine powder.

Then, into the pot went a cup of water, half a teaspoon of lemon juice and one teaspoon of salt.

The ground-up mixture of spices was added to the liquid stuff and the whole thing was brought to a good boil.

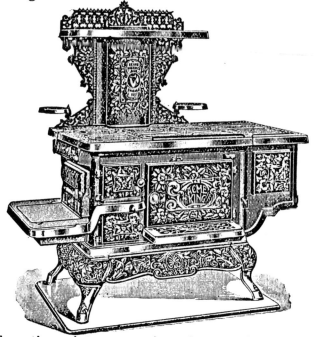

Then the mixture was just simmered for five minutes.

Seetha let a cup of this cool down enough so that Kumar could drink it, and he did. He forced down a full cup of that foul-tasting stuff.

In only an hour, his throat was better. He then finished off the rest of the remedy to keep the soreness from coming back.

—Jay Balachandran

THRUSH

Cure For Stepping on A Rusty Nail

A good cure for the infection that can result from stepping on a nail is kind of sickening, but it's supposed to work.

What you do is to soak your foot in horse urine, but that's just a little bit sickening compared to the next one I have.

It's for babies when they get a crust on their tongue. That condition is called Thrush and can be cured by having the baby suck on his wet diaper.

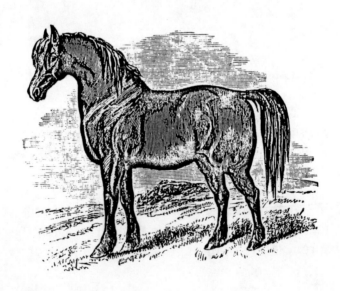

I'm not just real sure that all of these home remedies are what you'd call real good ideas.

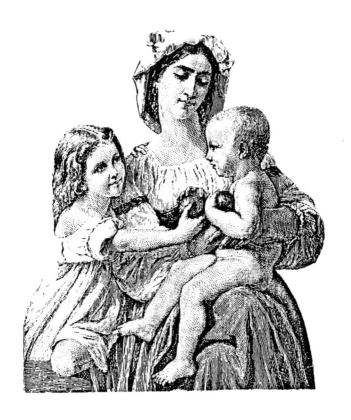

—Brent Mann

TONIC FOR SPRINGTIME

When my mother, Mary Lee, was a little girl she was given a "spring tonic" whether she needed it or not. It was supposed to keep her healthy all the rest of the year until the following spring.

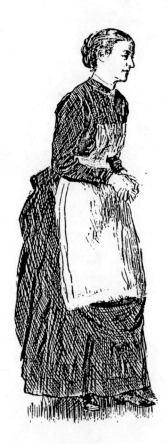

That tonic was made out of suphur and molasses. My grandmother would put in twice as much molasses as she would sulphur.

My mother said it tastes just awful, especially the suphur.

She never looked forward to the day she had to take that tonic, but my grandmother insisted. She even stood there and watched to be sure that her daughter drank the stuff instead of throwing it out.

—Meredith Lee

TOOTHACHES

Our family has an old remedy for a sore tooth.

What folks would do was to go into the woods and find a prickly ash bush. They would take one of the red berries, and put it on the tooth that hurt, and then bite down hard on it.

The berry was supposed to numb the tooth to make it quit hurting.

I don't know, but I 'spose they had to time their toothaches to the time when those prickly ash bushes had berries on them.

—Amanda Kitto

Wilma Dobson told me what she did when she got a toothache.

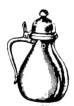 She'd dip a small piece of cotton in oil of cloves and press it tightly against the tooth so air would not get to it.

Then, she'd rush to the dentist.

—Lindsay Brodbeck

(141)

Not all remedies have to work. Some, like this one, are jokes.

Ed Miller developed a toothache one day and told his mother about it.

She thought hard about that situation and then told him that she remembered what her grandmother had told her.

"Ed, just fill your mouth up with water and sit on the stove 'til it boils."

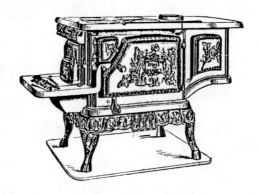

Of course, Ed didn't try that little remedy. I guess he just outlived his toothache.

I guess, too, that Ed's mother must have been pretty busy that day with other things.

—Matt Allen

TOOTHPASTE

For toothpaste my Grandma Lucille Moore used a mixture of salt and soda. She'd put it on a toothbrush like any other toothpaste and it work-ed real well.

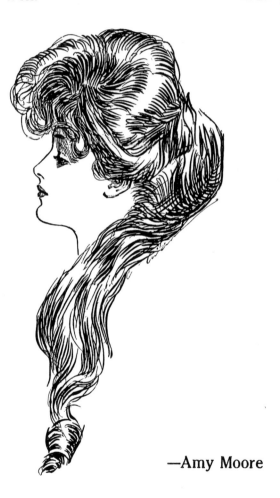

—Amy Moore

VINEGAR CURE-ALL

Vinegar was a home remedy for many things.

One thing folks used it for was to harden the skin.

But it did more. It was supposed to take the sting out of sunburn, to cure pimples, and cure impetigo.

It was good for the prevention of bruising, general cleansing, making the hair shine, and curing dry skin.

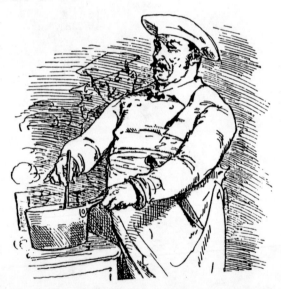

Besides all that, it was supposed to enable you to lose weight and could be rubbed directly on-to the spine to cure nervous conditions.

—Ken Hanson

WARTS

My mother's best friend, Cindy Fritz, used to get warts all of the time. At one time the poor girl had thirty-two warts on one hand.

One of her friends heard of a man who bought warts, so Cindy went to see him.

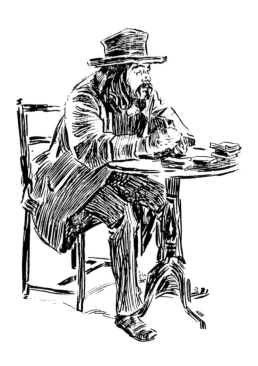

That strange man gave Cindy thirty-two pennies and told her to rub them on the warts, one on each wart.

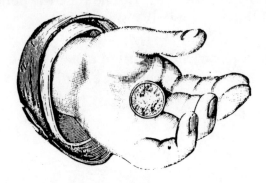

Then she was told she should go downtown in thirty-two days and buy one thing with all thirty-two pennies.

So, thirty-two days later she did just that and within a few days she woke up one morning and the warts were all gone!

—Bethany Haas

My grandmother, Leelavathi Parekh, lives here in Wisconsin. Where she grew up, there were some home remedies that could save a trip to the doctor's office. And here's a special one to get rid of warts.

They would take a string of hair from a horse's tail and tie it around the wart.

Every day they would tighten the hair until the wart fell off. Grandma claimed that this remedy really worked.

—Manish Maski

A remedy that my father's family would use for warts was the milkweed plant.

They would break the steam of the plant, open and collect the "milk" that would run out. That "milk" was supposed to be a good cure for warts.

—Sarah Smidt

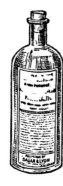

Cure for Planter's Warts

Dissolve thirty grams of salicyic acid in 1.2 oz. of flexible colladium. (You can get this at a drug store.)

Cover the warts until they go away.

—Jason Udelhofen

Years ago the Jonas family seemed to be cursed with warts.

Unfortunately, they didn't have the money to go to a doctor with their problem.

(147)

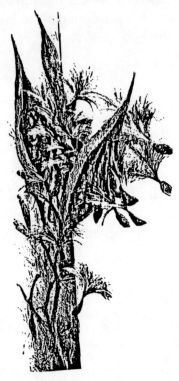

So the family fell back on an old cure that was a good one for where they lived near Muscoda, Wisconsin.

For near Muscoda there were lots of milkweeds.

They would just break the stem of the milkweed, and smear that thick white fluid from the stem onto their warts.

Daily treatment of this for about two weeks was all it took to make those warts disappear.

—Victor Jonas

WHOOPING COUGH

Whooping cough has ended up causing the death of many people by bringing on bronchitis, pneumonia, hemorrhages, or convulsions. It isn't a disease that one can be careless about.

And the worst part of it is that it is tougher on little children than it is on adults.

When Lee-Anne Sargent of Platteville was a little four-year-old, she came down with whooping cough.

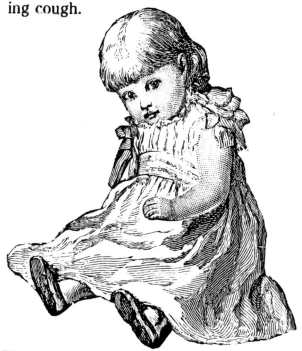

The medication the doctor was giving her wasn't seeming to do any good, so he told Lee-Anne's mother that she might as well try an old home remedy on her daughter.

(149)

He told her how to fix it, so that's what she did. She simmered an onion in a pan of water until it was soft and kind of mushy.

She then cut the onion into chunks and let it steep in a pan of hot water for a few minutes until the flavoring and odor of that onion had gotten into the water well.

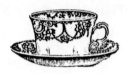 Lee-Anne had to drink a bunch of that onion tea. Her mother gave it to her in a cup from a doll's china set. That helped Lee-Anne to get by the taste of that onion tea a little bit, but it still tasted pretty bad.

Lee-Anne must have been convinced that the onion tea remedy worked on her, though, because she used it on her own children years later.

Onion tea can also be used on other illnesses related to congestion. It doesn't take very much. Just a couple of teaspoons every few hours is all that's necessary.

A person does have to be a little careful of onion tea. If you take too much of it, or you take it for too long, you can get diarrhea.

—Christy Sargent

WORMS

If I had lived back when they used a lot of home remedies, I sure would wish that I would never have a need to try this one.

It was a tea made out of sage that Grandma Lucille Moore used to cure a person of worms.

Grandma made it by using a teaspoon of sage and a cup of water. She'd boil that stuff up and as soon as it was brewed, the patient had to drink it.

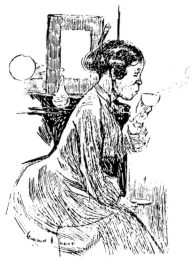

It all sounds pretty bad to me. I wouldn't want any part of it.

—Amy Moore

EPILOGUE

All those funny sounding things like skunk oil, saffron, and sassafras are not used much any more in Wisconsin in the 1990's. Nor do we think in terms of kerosene, walnut hulls, or creek bottom mud as being of medicinal value.

But Wisconsin folks back years ago used those things often and considered them to be important parts of their health care.

While the practice of medicine has changed, the love and care offered to children by their parents are still with us. But then, after all, that's a whole lot more important than goose grease or castor oil.

Need A Gift?

For

- **Shower** • **Birthday** • **Mother's Day** •
- **Anniversary** • **Christmas** •

Turn Page for Order Form
(Order Now While Supply Lasts!)

To Order Copies Of

Wisconsin's Early Home Remedies

Please send me _____ copies of **Wisconsin's Early Home Remedies** at $9.95 each. (Make checks payable to **QUIXOTE PRESS**.)

Name _____

Street _____

City _____ State _____ Zip _____

Send Orders To:
Quixote Press
R.R. #4, Box 33B • Blvd. Station
Sioux City, Iowa 51109

- -

To Order Copies Of

Wisconsin's Early Home Remedies

Please send me _____ copies of **Wisconsin's Early Home Remedies** at $9.95 each. (Make checks payable to **QUIXOTE PRESS**.)

Name _____

Street _____

City _____ State _____ Zip _____

Send Orders To:
Quixote Press
R.R. #4, Box 33B • Blvd. Station
Sioux City, Iowa 51109

If you have enjoyed this book, perhaps you would enjoy others from Quixote Press.

HUMOR:

Iowa's Roadkill Cookbook	B. Carlson	7.95
South Dakota's Roadkill Cookbook	B. Carlson	7.95
Missouri's Roadkill Cookbook	B. Carlson	7.95
Minnesota's Roadkill Cookbook	B. Carlson	7.95
Wisconsin's Roadkill Cookbook	B. Carlson	7.95
Illinois' Roadkill Cookbook	B. Carlson	7.95
How to Talk Midwestern	R. Thomas	7.95
A Field Guide to Missouri's Critters	B. Carlson	7.95
A Field Guide to Iowa's Critters	B. Carlson	7.95
A Field Guide to Illinois' Critters	B. Carlson	7.95

MISCELLANEOUS:

Memoirs of a Dakota Hunter	G. Scholl	9.95
Hitchhiking the Upper Midwest	B. Carlson	7.95
Me 'n Wesley		
(about homemade toys on the farm)	B. Carlson	9.95
Iowa, The Land Between the Vowels		
(farmboy tales)	B. Carlson	9.95
Iowa's Early Home Remedies	various	9.95
Illinois' Early Home Remedies	various	9.95
Missouri's Early Home Remedies	various	9.95
Underground Iowa		
(tales from under Iowa's soil)	B. Carlson	9.95
Underground Illinois	B. Carlson	9.95
Underground Missouri	B. Carlson	9.95
Early Iowa Schools	C. Johnston	9.95

OUTHOUSES:

Iowa's Vanishing Outhouse	B. Carlson	9.95
Missouri's Vanishing Outhouse	B. Carlson	9.95
The Dakota's Vanishing Outhouse	B. Carlson	9.95
Wisconsin's Vanishing Outhouse	B. Carlson	9.95
Minnesota's Vanishing Outhouse	B. Carlson	9.95
Illinois' Vanishing Outhouse	B. Carlson	9.95

ROMANCE:

Old Iowa Houses, Young Loves	B. Carlson	9.95

MIDWEST RIVERBOAT SERIES:

Jack King vs. Detective MacKenzie	N. Bell	9.95
River Sharks & Shenanigans	N. Bell	9.95
Lost & Buried Treasure of the Mississippi	Scholl/Bell	9.95
Romance on Board	H. Colby	9.95

MISSISSIPPI RIVER:

Mississippi River Po' Folk	P. Wallace	9.95
Strange Folks Along the Mississippi	P. Wallace	9.95
Mississippi River Cookin' Book	B. Carlson	11.95

GHOST STORIES:

Ghosts of the Miss. River, from Mpls. to Dub.	B. Carlson	9.95
Ghosts of the Miss. River, from Dub. to Keokuk	B. Carlson	9.95
Ghosts of the Miss. River, from Keokuk to S.L.	B. Carlson	9.95
Ghosts of Johnson County, Iowa	L. Erickson	12.95
Ghosts of Des Moines County, Iowa	B. Carlson	12.00
Ghosts of Scott County, Iowa	B. Carlson	12.95
Ghosts of The Amana Colonies, Iowa	L. Erickson	9.95
Ghosts of Polk County, Iowa	T. Welch	9.95
Ghosts of the Iowa Great Lakes	B. Carlson	9.95
Ghosts of Northeast Iowa	R. Hein et al.	9.95
Ghosts of the Black Hills	T. Welch	9.95
Ghosts of Door County, Wisconsin	G. Rider	9.95
Ghostly Tales of Southwest Minnesota	R. Hein	9.95
Ghosts of Rock Island County, Illinois	B. Carlson	12.95
Ghosts of the Coast of Maine	C. Schulte	9.95

LADIES OF THE EVENING:

Some Awfully Tame, But Kinda
  Funny Stories About:

—Early Iowa Ladies-of-the-Evening	B. Carlson	9.95
—Early Illinois Ladies-of-the-Evening	B. Carlson	9.95
—Early Wisconsin Ladies-of-the-Evening	B. Carlson	9.95
—Early Minnesota Ladies-of-the-Evening	B. Carlson	9.95
—Early Missouri Ladies-of-the-Evening	B. Carlson	9.95
—Early Dakota Ladies-of-the-Evening	B. Carlson	9.95

INDEX

A

B

C

D

E

F

G

H

I

J

K

L

M

N

O

P

Q

R

S

T

U

V

W

Y

(Year - Continued)